Help *and Hope* While You're Healing

A woman's guide toward wellness
while recovering from injury, surgery, or illness

Christine Carter

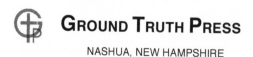

GROUND TRUTH PRESS

NASHUA, NEW HAMPSHIRE

Help and Hope *While You're Healing: A woman's guide toward wellness while recovering from injury, surgery, or illness*

Copyright © 2016 Christine Carter

Published by GROUND TRUTH PRESS
   P. O. Box 7313
   Nashua, NH 03060-7313

Editor: Bonnie Lyn Smith

Cover design: Michelle Fairbanks, Fresh Design

First printing 2016

Printed in the United States of America

This book is not intended as a substitute for the medical advice of physicians. The reader should regularly consult a physician in matters relating to his/her health and particularly with respect to any symptoms that may require diagnosis or medical attention.

Unless otherwise indicated, Scripture quotations are from *The Holy Bible, English Standard Version*® (ESV®). Copyright © 2001 by Crossway, a publishing ministry of Good News Publishers. Used by permission. All rights reserved.

Trade paperback ISBN-13: 978-0-9908303-3-7

Trade paperback ISBN-10: 0990830330

To _____

May you find help and hope while your healing.

With love,

_____

To my beloved husband and children—

For watching me at my worst and loving me anyway.
You have seen me through various injuries, surgeries, and
illnesses, and with patience and perseverance,
you have cared for me and helped me heal.

To all the amazing women who have endured far greater
circumstances, and yet find the strength and stamina to do
life with both grace and dignity—

You are my heroines.
I am in awe of your tenacity to push through your pain and
claim each day with the vigor and vigilance it takes to embrace
what you have and to use what you've got!

Any woman who has experienced injury, surgery, or illness has
a remarkable story,
so if you are reading this, please know—

I am inspired by yours.

CONTENTS

INTRODUCTION   1

1 I'LL MEET YOU THERE   5

A WORTHY WAIT   7

2 PREPARING FOR THE PAUSE   13

AREAS OF RESPONSIBILITY   14
WHO ARE YOUR HELPERS?   19
LIST OF HELPERS IN AREAS OF RESPONSIBILITIES   29

3 MANAGING THE PAIN   33

REFLECTION AND DETAILS OF YOUR GRATITUDE LIST   36
MANAGING THE PAIN—STAY OFF THE BRIDGE!   40
THE GARDEN OF GRATITUDE   45

4 REACH FOR YOUR PEOPLE   47

ON FRIENDS AND FEET WASHING   52

5 DISCOVER YOUR PASSION AND PURPOSE   57

WRITE OUT YOUR SPECIFIC PLAN FOR EACH PASSION   60
WHAT TO DO WHEN YOU'RE SICK   64

6 HONOR YOUR HEALING   67

WHAT ARE YOUR GIFTS?   71
HOW CAN YOU USE THESE GIFTS?   72
YOU ARE BEAUTIFUL   73

7 ADJUST YOUR LENS   77

SHIFT YOUR LENS TO A WIDER PERSPECTIVE   80

8 OWN IT, LAUGH A LITTLE, AND GET OUT!   85

FUNNY CAN BE FOUND ANYWHERE   89

9 PRAYER AND SPIRITUALITY   93

FOUR-STEP PRAYER   96
TO WALK IN FAITH...   99

10 A NEW DAY   103

BEAUTY BLOOMS IN HARD PLACES   106

11 AND ANOTHER THING...   109

YOUR PAIN IS A BEAUTIFUL REMINDER   111

ADDITIONAL NOTES   115

Introduction

IF I WERE you, I would want to know about the author of this book and how she was going to help me through my healing journey. I would want to learn what she has been through and how it relates to my circumstances. I would be curious about her experience and wonder if it would prove valuable in applying her wisdom and input to my own situation. At the very least, I would want to see a general health résumé detailing her qualifications and background, much like hiring someone for a job. You, my dear reader, deserve to know about me if you are willing to purchase this book and expect it to offer the help and hope I promise, right?

Let me introduce myself to you—through my very own injury, surgery, and illness résumé!

Christine Carter

Wife, mom, daughter, sister, aunt, cousin, friend, ministry leader, writer, and a self-proclaimed touchy-feely-super-sensitive goofball who loves to encourage people.

INJURIES

I broke my foot while running through the sprinkler with my kids and drove myself to the doctor with that broken foot.
(Bonus points?)

I broke my ankle running to first base while playing a mean game of wiffle ball with my family.
(I have since stopped running. Message received.)

I've stubbed my toe a million times.
(Does that count?)

SURGERIES

Foot Surgery: 2001

Double Mastectomy/Full Reconstruction/Full Hysterectomy (I call this my full feminine excavation): 2009

Dental Surgery (Five hours, 14 crowns. Thank you, anesthesia!): 2011

Lumpectomy (Parotid Tumor): 2013

Foot and Ankle Surgery (Broken Ankle/Fused Big Toe Joint): 2014

Foot Follow-Up (Took those nails out!): 2015

Upcoming Foot Surgery (Fuse other big toe joint): TBA

ILLNESSES

Among the various colds, flus, infections, and viruses that most humans acquire, I have survived the following debilitating afflictions:

Shingles

Pleurisy

Clostridium Difficile Colitis- otherwise known as C-Diff
(Recurring three agonizing times)

Gluten Intolerance
(Still searching for other causes of chronic illness I am currently experiencing)

*****

I have spent a good part of my life being healthy, but as you can see, I have some experience with injuries, surgeries, and illnesses, too.

While our experience with injury, surgery, or illness doesn't define who we are, it surely is one aspect we can honor and respect as part of our journey. It is from these hard-fought battles that I found inspiration to write this book.

Although you will find some posts from my blog site in this book, there are many additional articles at *The Mom Cafe* (themomcafe.com) on faith, motherhood, family, marriage, and healing/wellness. I would love for you to visit me there to learn more about me and my ongoing mission to offer encouragement, perspective, and inspiration in those significant areas of our lives.

Because I have experienced the difficult road toward healing and recovery many times, I wanted to share some insight to offer more depth and structure to your own recovery and to help you be ***well*** while you're healing. I know what you are going through, and I would be honored to walk alongside you.

Hold on, sister. You can do this.

Allow me to give you some ***help and hope while you're healing***.

1

I'LL MEET YOU THERE

H I, MY NEW friend. Right this very minute as I write these words, you are on my heart. I think about you so often—each one of you who will be reading this book. Please know that I will be praying this guide will help, prepare, nourish, and restore you through your suffering and lift you into a *purposeful plan* for this temporary season. I want nothing more than to encourage and meet you right where you are. I may not know the details of your particular situation, but I'm well aware of what it feels like to experience pain and the limitations from that pain.

If you are reading this, I can guess that you are hurting from an injury, surgery, or illness. I'm so sorry that you have to walk this road. I hope this book speaks to your heart and offers you hope and inspiration during this difficult time in your life.

Throughout this book, I will walk you through this journey of healing and offer you encouragement in those difficult areas you may find yourself in along the way. I will also share some of my own experiences with the hope of helping you maintain a healthy perspective and an understanding that you are not alone.

You can make it through this temporary time in your life. Much of it will be spent waiting to resume the life you once had.

> *You can make this passage through recovery a worthy*
> *wait; you can find purpose, fortitude, and perspective.*

It may seem like an impossible pursuit, but it *is* possible. I believe this challenging season can be an extraordinary experience. It will take some intention on your part—and a willingness to make this time count.

Are you ready?

We got this!

A Worthy Wait

I watched the kids swim while I sat in my wheelchair behind the glass in the lounge area, waiting...

...to pee.

*The kids had wheeled me into the recreation center and then proceeded to dart to the pool area like it was Disneyland, squealing with delight at the prospect of swimming for **fun** on a **school** night for my son's ninth birthday. I absolutely had to be there with my precious boy on his birthday. I needed to be a part of this, of something other than lamenting my pain and my restrictions at home. I had been stuck in a leg cast for eight weeks, and today was the day of liberation from that cast, only to receive a heavier brace on my leg to lug around for another month. As my leg throbbed from the transitional pull and push into something new, harsh, and heavy, I found, once again, that dreaded word:*

   waiting.

I had to pee. I always have to pee. This is not a good thing when you are unable to use one leg. It means all kinds of trouble. This ever-present need must be met often, and the "met" part is not easy. I was stuck in my wheelchair waiting while the kids soaked in a flow of water and joy.

My husband had dropped us all off on his way downtown to work on a property for a few hours. I sat and watched my kids have a glorious time together in the pool, thinking how wonderful it was they were enjoying each other so beautifully—a celebration of siblings on such a significant day. Oh, how I loved to see this! I felt my foot and ankle throbbing, so I kept pulling my leg up on the ledge of the window hoping to alleviate the pain. No such luck. I was hoping my husband would show up soon, so he could wheel me down the hallway and help me into the bathroom.

*By the time he arrived and I filled him in on the fun they'd been having, the pool was closing and it was time to go. He left me once again, this time to get the kids and supervise the showers and changing—**while I waited some more**.*

7

When we finally arrived home to have our cookie cake and wrap up the day, I sighed and murmured:

"I have been waiting to go to the bathroom all night!"

I hoisted myself onto the scooter and slowly clunked along, hitting doorways and hallway walls to get to the bathroom.

As I passed my chlorine-soaked birthday boy, he said,

"Mom, you're really getting good at waiting."

Then it hit me:

> I have been challenged in countless ways during this
> season of healing, and yet the greatest obstacle of all
> has been the waiting.

Waiting, waiting, waiting…

Waiting to heal. Waiting to sleep. Waiting to eat. Waiting to clean. Waiting to pee. Waiting to bathe. Waiting for laundry. Waiting for rides. Waiting to be an active mother and a true participant in life again. Waiting for the pain to stop along with this excruciating dependence for all my needs. Waiting for things I cannot control.

So much waiting.

And apparently, I have gotten better at it.

Hmm.

I kept thinking about what my sweet boy said to me, and I began to follow the waiting trail back for weeks, then months, then years. I traced the waiting through holding my breath in unfulfilled dreams and love's lingering hope. I recounted the many times I waited to hear back from music studios, job interviews, applications, submissions, schools, insurance settlements, doctors, lab tests, and diagnoses.

I remembered those longer waits, lasting years:

- *Seasons of wondering and hoping for what's to come*
- *Time periods of wishing things would change*
- *Days upon days of searching for the right man, the perfect home, and a miraculous medicine to make my daughter well*

I thought about parenting my two kids and how every single day is about waiting: leading and waiting, watching and waiting, teaching and waiting, hoping and praying anxiously that they "arrive" where I want them to be—both figuratively and literally.

Waiting through all those long gaps of time they are away from me, worrying if they are okay.

Waiting for one stage to be over and a new one to begin.

Waiting for them to poop, get their shoes on, respond when I call them, and finish their chores.

*Apparently, **so** much of my life is spent **waiting**.*

I am betting yours is too.

It ain't easy, is it? I know.

Waiting is a part of our every day, down to the detailed grit of overcrowded stores, traffic delays, phone calls on hold, school pick-up lines, and loading those apps.

I wonder how much time I have spent waiting in my 49 years of living. I wonder if I did anything worthwhile with all that time.

I'm hoping I did.

*Because if I ruminated on "what ifs," "when wills," or "come **on**s," I'm not sure I can say that I have had a productive waiting career.*

I think I wasted a lot of time stewing on those very things.

But waiting can be where our greatest growth occurs.

Think about it.

*I realized that time in the "stuck" (wondering, questioning, worrying, wishing, hoping) may actually bring new strength we never knew we had. That angst and anticipation, that frustration and surrendering, that ongoing challenge of acceptance and peace in the "now" surely can result in something great—like endurance, perseverance, maturity, wisdom, and learning the art of being fulfilled without being **full** or **filled**. It can teach us how to trust in God's will and not in our own. It can plunge us deep into surrender and reveal to us a new layer of fortification, sanctification, and even transformation.*

But it can be wrapped around hard barbed wire that makes it sting instead of sustain: bitterness, comparison, jealousy, discouragement, defeat, despair, frustration, anger, hopelessness.

Ouch.

*I've been there, and if you must wait long, **it's difficult to take**.*

Perhaps practice makes perfect. If we really dig in and open our eyes to discover the opportunities while we wait, maybe we can look back once we're finished waiting and see the glaring possibility that the waiting was meant to be, that it served a purpose.

Maybe.

> Although there are bridges that seem endless, taking us nowhere, we may in fact realize that they are really our training ground, not measured by the miles across, but rather by the strength of their architecture.

The bridge by itself can be quite beautiful if we intentionally design and build it. It could actually be exquisite—maybe even better than what we dreamed was on the other side. Within endurance and perseverance, we can discover extraordinary life lessons.

Maybe.

I dunno.

All I can say for sure is that I've gotten better at waiting.

*What if instead of declaring, "It was worth the wait," we were able to claim: "It was a **worthy** wait"?*

2
PREPARING FOR THE PAUSE

A T THIS TIME, you are either anticipating an upcoming surgery or you already have had your surgery and have found yourself down for the count, unsure of exactly how you will manage your limitations and adjust to this new normal. Perhaps you've had an injury or illness that has left you bedridden or immobile and you are facing the days ahead with no plan or preparation. This chapter offers you a chance to organize your plans *before* and/or *after* your surgery or time of convalescence.

As you begin this exercise, remind yourself several times that your life will experience a **pause**. A pause is merely a drop of time on your timeline, during which you will have to stop your usual routine for a temporary period. Keep that perspective, my friend. Pauses aren't permanent! Remind yourself of that often.

This preparation period is when it's time to get real. I know you might believe you can manage much like you did prior to this time of recovery—or perhaps you think you can simply get by for this temporary stretch of time. Maybe you can, but what if you can't?

Sometimes recovery is much more difficult than we expected. Despite our positive outlook, our bodies might voice otherwise. You will need support whatever your recovery process looks like. It's better to have a plan in place with the help you may need than to have no plan at all. It's important to have assistance and helping hands along the way—no matter your circumstances. If you are a mother, then you are likely already in high-gear preparations for childcare, home care, and carpools. If you live alone, I urge you to set up the home care you need, either by trusted friends or medical personnel. I believe it's better to be over-prepared than be stuck in pain and unable to carry out what you thought you would manage to do. I also believe having a plan and feeling prepared will help ease your anxiety about the aftermath of your surgery and the impact it may have on your life.

The details of your plan are unique to your specific needs, but there are basic areas of responsibility you must consider. Take some time to think through these questions. Then write down the contact people and assignments you have addressed in this task.

Areas of Responsibility

List all the major responsibilities you will need to put on your checklist. This checklist will identify tasks you need to either complete or delegate to someone else. If you are reading this because you suffer from chronic illness, much of this guide may be a useful resource for you on days you cannot manage your responsibilities on your own.

I have added the following areas:

1. Medical Preparations
2. Work
3. Housework/Meals/Groceries
4. Family
5. Parenting
6. Social Activities

You can write down all that you need to accomplish on the worksheets designated for each one. All these areas and tasks will be unique to your own circumstances, but I will share some examples to get you started. If you need an additional area of responsibility, I have another page for you to complete as well.

1. **Medical Preparations:** What do you need to do in order to prepare for your surgery? What needs to be in place if you become ill again?

Do you need to buy adaptive clothes? Medical equipment such as a scooter, walker, sling, wraps, lifts, or wheelchair?

Will you need your bathroom adapted to meet your physical needs?

What about bandages, cleaners, or ice packs?

Think through all you will need, and read any papers your doctor gave you to prepare for your operation.

Do you need to fill any prescriptions?

Do you need to schedule doctor appointments, physical therapy (PT) sessions, blood labs, procedures, follow-up visits, etc.?

Perhaps you need rides to many of these appointments.

Think through any preparation you need to have in place and what you anticipate you will need, both physically and medically, for your upcoming recovery period.

2. **Work:** This category is for any responsibilities you need to tend to that relate to your job.

Do you need to notify people of your time off?

Are there tasks you need to do prior to your absence? Calls to make, or papers to fill out?

Are there aspects of your job you must continue while you are recovering?

Are there contacts you need to communicate with on an ongoing basis?

Do you need to delegate assignments to coworkers, cancel meetings, reschedule deadlines, etc.?

3. **Housework/Meals/Groceries**: What needs to be done around the house?

Is there any yard work that will need tended to on an ongoing basis?

For however long you are off your feet and unable to clean the house, who will step in?

How about grocery shopping?

Can you stock up on things you will need and find someone to run to the store weekly for you?

Are you able to plan and prepare your meals and freeze them? Maybe you have a group of friends who are willing to make and deliver meals for you and your family while you recover.

4. **Family**: Do you have any responsibilities regarding your family, including your extended family?

Do you visit your father every week? Perhaps you help your sister out with her kids two days a week and need to help her find daycare for this time.

Who in your family can help you with your recovery needs? How can your husband or partner assist you through this?

Maybe you need to contact your ex to figure out transportation and childcare throughout the week.

Whatever pertains to any family members, events, and activities that may be coming up in the future, check your calendar and make sure you are not forgetting important dates. Maybe there are birthdays ahead and you would like to send cards in advance.

5. **Parenting:** If you're a mom, then you know this one deserves its own category!

I'm guessing your task list might be loaded with things to do, depending on how many kids you have and their ages.

What appointments are ahead?

Do your children need rides to school?

Do you have little ones in need of someone coming to the house to care for them every day?

Do you need to stock up on diapers? Medicine?

Perhaps a new season is coming and the kids have outgrown their clothes.

Any last-minute shopping for clothes, sports equipment, books for school, Christmas presents?

Who's going to help with the laundry?

Do you need assistance with your children's extracurricular activities?

6. **Social Activities:** This area is for all the extra activities you are involved in aside from work and family.

Are you in any church ministries, book clubs, sport organizations, school PTA meetings, or support groups?

Think through all your hobbies and interests and where you spend your free time. Then write down what needs to be cancelled, rescheduled, or delegated to someone else.

I would suggest going through your calendar and skimming the weeks of the previous months to ensure you haven't forgotten anything—and surely jump ahead through the next few months too! You will also need to look through your schedule in the months to come and make decisions now to cancel or ask others to take your place (if it's a commitment or role you have). As hard as it may be to cancel something months in advance, when the time comes, you will be incredibly relieved that you did!

> *I strongly encourage you to go past your planned date of full recovery.*

Reentrance into the world needs to be slow and easy. I can't tell you how many times I assumed I would be ready to jump back into my normal active life, but when that time came around, I wasn't even close to being able to participate. I know you think you can do it, but please assume you will not be fully recovered for at least one month **after** the expected date of complete health. Even if you can ease back into your life around that time, you will need to pace yourself according to your strength and ability to be truly active in all your roles.

> *You will not be able to do it all at once, I promise.*

I know all too well about this mistake and the reality of our physical limitations versus our best intentions. You will need acclimation time as your body adjusts to entering back into your routines, activities, and schedule. You won't have the strength or the stamina to dive into everything all at once. Slowly add one thing, and then see how you feel. If you handled it well, then add one more thing. How'd that go? Maybe you can go ahead with half a day of work. Perhaps you can carry that one light load of laundry now. If you are able to drive, maybe you can attend a meeting or go back to church.

You simply can't do it all at once. ***Please*** ease your way back. It's the only way you will be able to remain healthy and protect your freshly healed injury, surgical area, or body after illness.

Who Are Your Helpers?

As you are recording all your tasks, you should be thinking of the people who will be assisting you with all these responsibilities. After you identify tasks in each of your major areas, you will have space to write down the name and phone number of whoever will be responsible for each task. If you are able to choose people ahead of time to serve you in your recovery, your healing will go much smoother, and it will surely be less stressful!

It would also be helpful to you (and others who are helping you) if you created a master contact list to refer to whenever needed. You can organize this list according to the main areas of responsibilities. You may want to make several copies of it. (Tape it to your fridge!)

Perhaps you had an accident and became injured or fell ill with no warning.

> *You can still work through all these areas and get your life back in order now.*

I'm sure you feel like you have lost all control, so this exercise may help you feel empowered once again to make these decisions and ask your helpers to tend to the tasks that haven't been completed.

This part of preparation is very difficult to work through, as you must release control of so much. For those fiercely independent individuals, this will be a very challenging time for you. You won't have meals made the way you want them. You won't have clean clothes folded the way you fold them. You won't operate your daily life at all like you used to. You may feel incredibly powerless in this place. And frustrated. And even depressed. I know I was.

It's hard, girls. So, **so** hard. Some of you may need help bathing, getting dressed, or wiping your butt. You will feel helpless, small, humiliated, angry, and hopeless. Here's where you need to surrender your control, power, and sensibility more than any other time in your life. You must learn to **let go**.

> *This is the time to accept that your life will look very,*
> *very different for a while.*

This isn't the normal, healthy, vibrant, and strong you. You may hate every minute of this, but you can choose to control your emotions and mind with your own strength and perspective. I don't know about you, but I sure think the strongest, most inspiring people on this planet are the ones who have had an accident or illness and have lost their "normal" lives—only to pick themselves up and boldly transition to living a new one—permanently.

Permanently. How would you feel if you found yourself right where you are for***ever***? Thinking along these lines always helped me to gain perspective.

"This is temporary." This will be your mantra, okay?

Say it with me:

> *This is temporary. This is temporary. This is temporary.*
> *This is temporary.*

Okay, so with that said, this temporary part of life is pretty awful. You must allow people to help you make it better.

This is the time to let others serve you, especially if you are usually the one who serves. You must find peace in accepting this time to be a season of **receiving**. There will be opportunities for you to give, but now is the chance for you to rest and take in the gifts of others. Find fulfillment in knowing that this choice will bless the people in your life who want to help care for you. You need to surrender in this regard; be glad you have people in your life who want to help you! Remind yourself that if the roles were reversed, you would be more than willing to help another friend out if they were in need.

> *Allow people to come into your life and bless you with*
> *what they can offer.*

Simply feel the gratitude, and *do not feel the pressure to reciprocate.* There will surely come a time when you will have that opportunity. Take heart, my friend. Know that this is the time for you to be lifted, carried, loved, and supported.

You know how good it feels to help someone out, right? Let others have the same pleasure in helping **you** out this time around.

Okay, then.

Now, go make your lists!

The next few pages are your checklists. Scribble on them with all your needs, and check them off as you go. Bring your book with you wherever you go, and use it as an ongoing reference to help keep your life organized!

MEDICAL PREPARATIONS		
Check	**Task**	**Helper/Contact**
☐		
☐		
☐		
☐		
☐		
☐		
☐		
☐		
☐		
☐		
☐		
☐		

WORK		
Check	**Task**	**Helper/Contact**
☐		
☐		
☐		
☐		
☐		
☐		
☐		
☐		
☐		
☐		
☐		
☐		
☐		

HOUSEWORK/MEALS/GROCERIES		
Check	Task	Helper/Contact
☐		
☐		
☐		
☐		
☐		
☐		
☐		
☐		
☐		
☐		
☐		
☐		
☐		

FAMILY		
Check	Task	Helper/Contact
☐		
☐		
☐		
☐		
☐		
☐		
☐		
☐		
☐		
☐		
☐		
☐		
☐		

PARENTING		
Check	**Task**	**Helper/Contact**
☐		
☐		
☐		
☐		
☐		
☐		
☐		
☐		
☐		
☐		
☐		
☐		
☐		

SOCIAL ACTIVITIES		
Check	Task	Helper/Contact
☐		
☐		
☐		
☐		
☐		
☐		
☐		
☐		
☐		
☐		
☐		
☐		
☐		

Check	Task	Helper/Contact
☐		
☐		
☐		
☐		
☐		
☐		
☐		
☐		
☐		
☐		
☐		
☐		
☐		

List of Helpers in Areas of Responsibilities

Medical Preparations Helpers

Name: _____ Phone: _____

Name: _____ Phone: _____

Name: _____ Phone: _____

Name: _____ Phone: _____

Work Helpers

Name: _____ Phone: _____

Name: _____ Phone: _____

Name: _____ Phone: _____

Name: _____ Phone: _____

Housework/Meals/Groceries Helpers

Name: _____ Phone: _____

Name: _____ Phone: _____

Name: _____ Phone: _____

Name: _____ Phone: _____

Family Helpers

Name: _____ Phone: _____

Name: _____ Phone: _____

Name: _____ Phone: _____

Name: _____ Phone: _____

Parenting Helpers

Name: _____ Phone: _____

Name: _____ Phone: _____

Name: _____ Phone: _____

Name: _____ Phone: _____

Social Activities Helpers

Name: _____ Phone: _____

Name: _____ Phone: _____

Name: _____ Phone: _____

Name: _____ Phone: _____

_____ **Helpers**

Name: _____ Phone: _____

Name: _____ Phone: _____

Name: _____ Phone: _____

Name: _____ Phone: _____

3
MANAGING THE PAIN

I KNOW YOU are hurting. Perhaps you are in so much pain, it's almost unbearable to hold this book in your hands and focus on the words I'm offering you.

I understand that pain.

Pain has great power, doesn't it?

Our physical pain can translate easily to emotional pain. Our suffering can saturate our perspective and thought life. It can ignite incredible mental anguish. When our bodies are in crisis mode, our thoughts and feelings often follow suit.

Pain has a way of twisting and turning our well-being and taking over every aspect of who we are.

Don't let it.

You can either surrender to the pain, causing a downward spiral of despair and defeat, or take control of your thoughts with relentless strength and inspiration. It's so easy to allow pain to take over your existence and keep you captive in a prison of survival. This can go on for days and days while you tremble and moan, crying out in despair. I have been there, sweet friend. I know that pain and that power all too well. I was stuck in that awful pit and finally figured out how to climb out despite the pain—and in spite of my situation. You can too. You **must** take the power back. Your mind can do that. You have a choice.

> *Every day you manage to bear this burden, you can control your thought life by shifting the focus from your pain to your praise.*

Take control of your thoughts and feelings right now.

Make a gratitude list. Write down every person, passion, or purpose you are thankful for in your life. Think of the way you spend your time. Brainstorm all the elements in your life that bring you joy and fulfillment. Envision a big-picture landscape when looking down at your life, and then narrow your focus to search the details: your family, your kids, your friends, your volunteer roles, your career, your community, your faith, the organizations you belong to, the experiences you enjoy, the memories you treasure, etc.

Whatever brings you **joy**, *write it down*!

Now narrow down those details even more. Describe what you love about these treasures in your life. Think through how they have brought you fulfillment. Has that changed? I am guessing that many of those elements have not changed; therefore, they still stand to bring you happiness in some way. Maybe you aren't able to *actively enjoy* them right now, but reflecting on them will remind you how very important they are to you, consequently filling you with gratitude.

Can you reflect on the detailed moments and experiences you have had? Imagine past memories, the ones that took your breath away with happiness. Dive into why you love these significant moments and people. Soak in the joy it brings you as you pour your thoughts onto the page and allow the feelings to follow.

Perhaps you can add more to this list. Maybe you want to pace yourself and stick with your first person or experience now and continue with the next one later. You can build an ongoing list of positive aspects and focus on one or two when you need to pull yourself away from your pain.

I have found this exercise to be very helpful in managing my pain. It will keep you from becoming discouraged and defeated, as you stretch the focus outside your pain and intentionally center your thoughts on those important parts of your life. This will help you maintain a healthy perspective and emotional stability.

When we experience debilitating pain, our outlook becomes blurry and our framework falls apart. We need to keep securing our perspective with all the supporting borders of goodness we still hold in our lives. Being intentional with your thoughts and revisiting all those moments and people you love will keep you anchored and will prevent you from giving into the pain completely.

> *There are also times when a good hard cry is what you need.*

Release the pressure of all that pent-up pain, and allow yourself to feel every bit of the mental, emotional, and physical anguish you are experiencing. You can have a heck of a pity party in this place, I know! Do it, but be sure you don't stay at the party too long. It can trap you and hold you captive if you do. Once you explore that deep despair and feel every raw emotion, you must come back up to the surface and focus on those positive places you identified. I found this lifted me into a different mindset every time I felt hopeless and helpless in the pain I was experiencing. I used all my strength to control my thinking and return to my gratitude list after every pity party I threw.

Reflection and Details of Your Gratitude List

Example

<u>My husband</u>

I think back to our wedding day when he first saw me in my gown. I cried, and because I had a sinus infection, snot poured from my nose as he kept handing me tissue after tissue. This scene always feels prophetic to me. After 15 years, my beloved continues to care for me in that same way. I am **so** grateful for him.

1. _____

_____

_____

_____

_____

2. _____

_____

_____

_____

_____

3. _____

_____

_____

_____

_____

4. _____

_____

_____

_____

_____

5. _____

_____

_____

_____

_____

6. _____

_____

_____

_____

_____

7. _____

_____

_____

_____

_____

8. _____

_____

_____

_____

_____

9. _____

_____

_____

_____

_____

10. _____

_____

_____

_____

_____

Managing the Pain—Stay off the Bridge!

I'm not a stranger to managing pain. I have had four surgeries in five years. Each one of them left me in pretty bad shape.

Pain has so much power.

There is a slippery bridge from physical pain to mental anguish. I try not to step on it. I know what's on the other side, and it's uglier than the physical pain. Have you been there?

Ah, the evil snares of pain. It can take over your every thought—and every minute—if you let it. But I give in. Sometimes.

I can't do a darn thing to control the pain, other than wait it out. It's healing, I say. Bit by bit. I can't question the why or how long because that leads me to that bridge. I can't think about it too long...or that bridge appears and lures me to the other side.

It's exhausting.

Attempting to live on one leg doesn't work too well with my intentions. I'm guessing it doesn't work too well in anyone's life, really.

Try it. I dare you.

Get yourself a glass of water.

Pull yourself off the couch and hop a dozen times to make it over to your scooter while grabbing at the coffee table for balance. Then twist the scooter a half dozen times while lifting it to place it in the direction you need to go while balancing on one leg. Wind around backpacks and furniture, causing you to stop and lift the scooter up and redirect it over and over again to get to the kitchen. When you reach into the fridge, be careful not to fall or lose your balance because you no longer have the security of wheels that slide to hold you in place. It takes a leg of steel to steady yourself and jump from the fridge to the counter every time you want a drink. And God forbid you try to clean out that fridge...all the while balancing on one leg. Don't take out those heavy casserole dishes, or you will surely pay for it.

Twenty minutes later, with sweat pouring from your face, you realize it isn't worth the battle to calm your mental need to find order and control. So you work your way back to the couch, where it seems you belong.

Another day.

Stuck.

You lie there, constantly trying to pull yourself up with your wrists that are so sore you can barely put pressure on them. They are tired of leveraging your weight over and over again. You simply cannot get comfortable. Parts of your body ache and tingle and spit at you with pain.

Then, of course, there is the pulsating original pain. This dominates your body as it scratches at your nerves with sheer fire; you catch your breath and wait it out until it turns into a slow hum of tiny knives and throbbing hammers that taunt here and there. Your calf wants some attention, too, so it clenches its fists, and you can't do even one thing to stretch it out.

So it twists tighter…

And tighter.

You want to eat at the cast until it tears off, so you can scratch and gnaw and claw at the scabs and wounds until they hear you.

"STOP!!"

You reach for a sip of your water…but you are reminded again of how weak your upper body has become. It's nearly impossible to lift a simple cup, and you decide to save the strength for those times you must climb up stairs, hoist yourself on and off toilets, or balance yourself into and out of slippery bathtubs.

41

You can't put your wounded foot down on the couch because every placement you try releases more pain from the touch of pressure, so you hold it in the air.

Try this way—and that. Lift here and there, tug the blanket, push the pillow, and pull the cushion until you finally fall asleep, restless, all the while knowing that this vicious limb will wake you with a penetrating seizure of explosive fireworks.

This is a tiny piece of my living.

So I wait…it out.

Tonight I started to let it get to me. Deep down…to that place.

You know that fragile place that is fenced off with all our faith and functioning and fortitude?

It's guarded well throughout our lives, but there are some storms that take that fence down.

I felt it collapsing into a slippery bridge beckoning me toward it.

Pain can do that. It can break you down to that place of crumbling despair and rage.

I exclaimed, "NO!! I won't let you take me down!"

And I flashed back in my mind to hours earlier…I envisioned it all.

> *I watched my daughter come home from school and get straight to her work as she worried about four more tests this week and a project. She organized her papers and folders at the table, and I watched her, so focused and driven to do her very best. I asked her all about her day and told her how proud I was of her choices, amazing motivation, and commitment to her studies.*
>
> *She worked for hours showing me her completed project with a smile. She ate and was off to her swim practice. She came back*

and told me she did really well with a very hard training, and there was that glow I so adore but don't see often. She believed in her progress for the first time in weeks. Her eyes were red and her hair soaked as she emptied all her equipment. She looked exhausted—but happy and proud.

I squealed with delight over the news and told her once again how incredibly proud I was of how hard she has worked all year. I was amazed at her determination and unbelievable stamina.

We snuggled together while watching football, and she sighed and squeezed into me with her whispering, "I love you, Mom." I pulled her in tighter and started to kiss her all over her face as she giggled.

"You're my favorite girl in the whole wide world," I said.

She was exhausted. She knew she couldn't make it another minute, so up she went to bed. I climbed the stairs behind her and crawled down the hall to hoist myself up on her way-too-high bed. I rolled over to throw my good leg over her body and pulled her in tight.

Lying with my daughter attempting to snuggle as best I could with my one working leg around her, somehow we managed.

I ignored the pain; I defied it by embracing the moment. I felt her sweet breath on my face as we spoke that special mother-daughter love. I told her for the 400th time today how proud I was of her and how amazing I think she is, as I repeated all the reasons why once again.

This is where my mind shall go—oh, the joy!

Oh, the love! I inhale it in, as I soften with such beauty to behold. I decide to stay there instead of stepping onto that bridge.

I am blessed.

I pray for those who are in pain. I know many of you. I think I learned the greatest way to defeat that monster is what I did—and continue to do. Claim the beauty in your life. Relive it. Soak in it. Let it take you out of that taunting place where you fall deeper into despair. Let it lift you into tears of joy and gratitude. Bask in it. Revel in it!

Perhaps the pain will live on, but your newfound strength will surpass it, and joy will defeat it, and love—oh, the love...

The love will outlast it.

I will not step onto that bridge. I have too much beauty to behold...

On this side.

Don't you?

Managing the Pain

The Garden of Gratitude

When your world is spinning...
Fast and furious off its axis,
Parts and pieces flying all around...
Unsettled and stirring in the fury
Of perhaps a storm hit hard unknowingly.

When your earth's breaking apart...
Crumbling into parts and pieces,
Scattering thoughts swirling with the dirt
As though gravity has lost its pull,
You become unbound,
Untethered to your truths.

Dig your heels in the ground,

Tend to the garden...

Of Gratitude.

There's fertile soil there
To plant the seeds of strength
Where perspective blooms
And fortitude blossoms,

Where restoration and transformation give way
To affirmation.

Your world may be turning
Recklessly and restlessly,
But your footing can be found
When you dig your heels in the ground

And tend to the garden...

Of Gratitude.

There are hidden treasures lying there
Beneath the spoils and toils of trouble.
Dig deeper to anchor your weight in...
You'll discover their power
And unearth the jewels of joy.

Let the richness soothe your mind;
Taste the sweetness of its pleasure.
Hold on tight. Grasp the light
Beyond the whirling winds.

Plant your peace...

In the budding ground
Underneath your feet.

And as your world spins...

~Bask in the bouquet from your garden~

Of Gratitude.

4
REACH FOR YOUR PEOPLE

DURING THIS TIME in your life, you need support more than anything. We women tend to think we can manage it all on our own. We are strong and independent and often tackle life's obstacles and challenges with our "*I got this*" mentality. I understand this all too well. You may still feel like you can handle it all and manage it from your recovery bed or couch, limping along, trudging through life's tasks as best you can. And yet, wouldn't it be easier if you asked people for help?

Maybe you realize you are incapable of doing it all. You are absolutely convinced you need extra arms, legs, drivers, meals, housekeepers, and caretakers to come in and care for those areas in your life you simply cannot handle. I suppose it depends on your circumstances and how difficult your recovery is.

One thing I'm sure of is that we tend to take on more than we should. This does ***not*** fare well in contributing to our healing process.

Friends, this is your season to be at rest as much as you can, and there are people in your life who are willing to step in; they are waiting for your call.

I remember before I had one of my surgeries, I thought I could handle the recovery on my own. I told my friends I was good to go, no need for meals or anything to assist in the post-surgery recovery. That very day after the surgery, lying on the couch, I began to sob and texted my friend with this claim:

"I can't do this. PLEASE HELP!"

I'm so grateful for people who can swoop in with their arms stretched open to carry our burdens when we simply can't handle the load. Do you have those people? That band of girlfriends who would dive into any pit to help you climb out? Perhaps you have that one best friend who would be at your doorstep in an instant if there were a need. Or maybe a sibling, parent, aunt, or coworker is a trusted companion you can always count on. Are you affiliated with a support group, church fellowship, or any group that could offer you help?

> *The people in your life will be a huge factor in your recovery. You simply must allow yourself to be served by them.*

Another important gift our people can give us during this time is the gift of simply offering an ear, a shoulder, a hug. When we are laid up, there is much loneliness and isolation. I know. This is the time to reach out to your trusted people and ask for a visit or a phone call. Perhaps you can even send simple texts asking for prayer or encouragement. When we are in pain and alone and are facing time ahead without our usual activities and schedules, it can be incredibly discouraging and defeating. We may not feel like reaching out, but we must. Our people will not know we are in need unless we tell them. Life pulls us in different directions, and it is up to us to inform others of our requests, needs, and troubles. If you are feeling lonely and unable to manage your circumstances, please reach out to at least one person you trust. In doing so, you will find relief and encouragement in the connection and assistance. Allow people to help care for you and tend to your needs. Remember that this **blesses** them as much as it will bless you.

Let go of those reciprocal expectations, guilt, and apologies for inconveniencing others. That is nonsense. Repeatedly remind yourself that you would serve your people in their times of need without any expectations or reciprocation. This isn't about keeping score or tabs on what they do for you and what you must give back. Allow yourself to be served by people who love and care for you. This is your time to receive. There will be many opportunities ahead to switch places and help someone else.

Who are your trusted people? With whom can you be completely honest, and on whom can you depend without feeling the weight of reciprocation? Reach out to them. Be specific about what you need so they can better serve you. There may be certain friends who would be great listeners. Other friends might sit and pray with you. Still others could bring a movie and popcorn over, while another friend may surprise you with takeout and good old-fashioned girl talk. You need your people! Don't isolate in despair. Reach out to those you trust and can count on for meeting your needs.

List your trusted confidantes and how they can each meet your needs:

Confidante: _____

Your Need:

_____

_____

_____

_____

_____

Confidante: _____

Your Need:

_____

_____

_____

_____

_____

Confidante: _____

Your Need:

_____

_____

_____

_____

_____

Confidante: _____

Your Need:

_____

_____

_____

_____

_____

Confidante: _____

Your Need:

_____

_____

_____

_____

_____

Confidante: _____

Your Need:

_____

_____

_____

_____

_____

On Friends and Feet Washing

I have been blessed with an amazing amount of true and unconditional friendships throughout my life: so many dear souls who have embraced, loved, and cared for me during times of suffering. So many women have loved me exactly as I am, where I am. They have accepted all my quirks and goofball antics as they laugh as much as cry with me. Oh, I can't tell you how grateful I am for so many wonderful people God has placed in my life!

Friendships are God's way of taking care of us.

I pray I give back as much as I receive.

Genuine friends are there for you in times of crisis. They not only show up, but they dive in. Each beautiful and precious act of service shines light into our lives. Through all the valuable and cherished memories I have of loved ones stepping in to help, there are those rare and raw moments of sacrifice that touch my heart so deeply: those times when a friend has gone above and beyond what they would be called to do, only because they love me. Those are the moments when I realize that laying down your life for a friend brings deeper meaning and an entirely new view of true friendship.

There are so many opportunities around us to serve our loved ones, friends, and even those we don't know well—or don't know at all. But how many of us truly tune in? It takes a mighty heart to look beyond our own lives and give of ourselves in such a way that challenges our comfort zones. I want to stretch, push, and strengthen this very part of giving.

I want to place my priorities where they are most needed—not where I most need them.

One summer a friend did exactly that for me. It was a simple and precious act, and yet it was profound and sacrificial, rendering such love that it brought me to tears.

I was going through some turmoil in my family life, and she was well aware I was both depleted and hurting. She encouraged me to go to the pool so our kids could swim while we soaked in some sun and drowned in our laughter—because with her I always laugh. I agreed to her request knowing full well that it was the best medicine and would help pull me out of my own stuff.

*This friend of mine is one of those friends who is **always** so perfectly dressed from head to toe. She is gorgeous. Every single time I see her (which is very often), she looks amazing, adorned with adorable outfits, cool accessories, and perfectly matching jewelry to boot. Head to toe. (But don't be misled; she is as real as they come.)*

I, on the other hand, live in sweat socks and gym shoes. Gym shorts and tank tops. My hair is always in a messy bun or ponytail with minimal everything just to get by. I am far from modeling the latest fashion and fail miserably at presentation. She loves me anyway and often helps me with my hair and outfits with a glorious, unconditional slathering of love.

One thing I deplore is my feet. They are wretchedly neglected because they ferment in my sweat socks and gym shoes all day long. My feet are often in pain as I have bone-on-bone grinding in my joints, which I have lived with for years. I cannot wear sandals, flip-flops, or any cute shoes for that matter. It's hard to have stylish outfits with gym shoes and sweat socks. It simply is what it is, and I'm okay with that, although it doesn't stop me from longing to wear some spiffy shoes and have pretty feet.

She knows all this.

When we get to the pool and find a place to sit down, I take off my gym shoes to air out my hot, stinky feet. My friend opens her bag to pull out her pedicure supplies. She reaches over to take my foot, gently pulling off my sock and exposing the nastiness there. I immediately pull it back and squeal with disgust, "What are you doing?!" She reclaims my foot while she gently persuades, "I am giving you a much-needed pedicure."

I stare at her in total disbelief while she fiddles through her polish, cleaners, and lotions to find her filer and starts working on my neglected toenails.

She sees absolutely nothing wrong with this act, despite me being horrified.

This perfectly pristine and ever-so-elegant woman has my smelly, sweaty, fungus-ridden foot in her beautifully manicured hands—and she is focused only on loving me.

Each nasty toe at a time.

Above and beyond.

To her, it was simply giving me comfort and pampering in her own unique and compassionate way.

1 John 3:16

By this we know love, that he laid down his life for us, and we ought to lay down our lives for the brothers.

I am deeply aware of and in awe of the power of this verse. There are moments of sacrifice that resonate in our lives in the literal sense. When we give so much of ourselves to another person, we truly lay down our lives in various ways.

And yet, there are those surprisingly simple, yet profound, acts of service that really "get me" right where I am:

A pedicure at the pool.

Perhaps God didn't picture it this way...

Or maybe He did.

Because I could have sworn that Jesus washed my feet that day.

John 13:14-15

"If I then, your Lord and Teacher, have washed your feet, you also ought to wash one another's feet. For I have given you an example, that you also should do just as I have done to you."

5

Discover Your Passion and Purpose

During this period of time when you are unable to carry on your normal, active life, you need to have something to do with your time as you recover. You may already have grand plans to get "*a ton of stuff done*" while you are laid up. Let me warn you: **This will not be the case, sweetie.** Often, your time will be spent asleep or managing your daily tasks like eating, drinking, going to the bathroom, and bathing. It's incredible how much time that will take out of your day. I don't want to discourage you from finding purpose in this time and being productive. I believe it is *so* important that we find this time to be both productive and purposeful, but I also want you to be realistic about your intentions. Remind yourself that you may not master or complete all the goals included within this chapter—*but*, you will have brainstormed some great ideas that you can pursue further when you recover.

While you are recuperating, you must understand that rest is most important, but restlessness will go along with it! You may feel like you aren't getting anything done, but healing is the most important goal of all. And healing doesn't appear productive—it rather looks like sleeping, taking medicine, and trying to manage the pain every day. This may not *feel* productive, only because you can't track your cell growth, bone strength, wounds healing, or immune system's ability to fight off illness like you can check off a to-do list.

It's rather frustrating to not have documentation of all that your body has accomplished every day while you appear to be doing nothing at all. The physical body is a miraculous and complex structure that often is overlooked. We tend to focus solely on our task lists and what we do outside our bodies, rather than appreciate all that work this intricate system must do in order to recuperate and function properly. If you struggle with needing to get stuff done, much like I did, you should reassure yourself every day that you in fact accomplished more than you know. We'll talk more about healing in the next chapter, but I didn't want to mislead you into thinking that you will be super-industrious during this time.

You may have severe limitations on certain pursuits you are passionate about. Those will have to wait, but you still have a working **mind** and a passionate **heart**, and that is enough to pursue many ideas.

Create a master plan, and organize goals for that plan.

What do you love?

Have you always wanted to explore a certain hobby but never found the time to learn the craft?

Perhaps there are stacks of books on your shelf you've been meaning to read. Does your library have educational audiobooks someone can bring you to listen to while you rest?

Maybe you have wanted to organize a fundraiser online for a friend in need of financial help, or perhaps you want to *finally* write to that old friend you haven't contacted in years.

Do you have pictures you've been wanting to organize and put into a scrapbook?

How about an online course you can take that is self-paced?

Maybe there are specific documentaries you have always wanted to watch but never had the time.

Whatever you can do with your mind and whatever *is* working in your physical body—*now* is the time to do it! You have hours to yourself, and you can turn this time into a productive and purposeful season, despite your limitations. In doing so, your focus will shift toward other ideas and tasks to accomplish instead of being stuck in your stillness and slow-moving moments of the day. This will give you newfound energy and inspiration to wake up every day and produce something, accomplish anything, make this time ***count***!

You may be feeling like this season of "stuck" and "still" will be a waste of time because you can't live according to your usual "normal."

> *This is a temporary pause, and if you are intentional about this space on your timeline, you can make it matter.*

You can dare to dream and pursue interests you never had the time for before. When your healing is complete, you can look back on this time and realize you were able to discover or experience something you never would have, had you not been out of commission for a while. What a wonderful way to be able to use this time for good!

Let's brainstorm your passions and plan your pursuits!

Remember: This list is a guide for you to follow when you are able. **When you are *able*.** Don't plan goals that are unrealistic or too burdensome. Make them manageable and simple. These ideas should be fulfilling and meaningful.

Write Out Your Specific Plan for Each Passion

Example

I've always wanted to read more about missionaries.

1. Search online for missionary biographies at my local library.
2. Check out one or two books that look interesting.
3. Have a friend pick up the books for me this week.
4. Try to read one chapter a day.

PASSIONS AND PLANS MASTER LIST

PASSION: _____

PLAN:

1. _____

2. _____

3. _____

4. _____

5. _____

PASSION: _____

PLAN:

1. _____

2. _____

3. _____

4. _____

5. _____

PASSION: _____

PLAN:

1. _____

2. _____

3. _____

4. _____

5. _____

PASSION: _____

PLAN:

1. _____

2. _____

3. _____

4. _____

5. _____

PASSION: _____

PLAN:

1. _____

2. _____

3. _____

4. _____

5. _____

Discover Your Passion and Purpose

PASSION: _____

PLAN:

1. _____

2. _____

3. _____

4. _____

5. _____

PASSION: _____

PLAN:

1. _____

2. _____

3. _____

4. _____

5. _____

What to Do When You're Sick

*I am not a good "sick person." I moan and groan and complain that I need to "get things done." I **absolutely hate** to cancel activities in my life. I stagger around the house attempting to push productivity as I force myself forward without forfeiting the loss of time. I begrudgingly reflect on the dinner gathering I was supposed to host, the Sunday School class that I should have taught, and the important meeting I couldn't make.*

Oh, woe is me...

I consider any "downtime" to be a waste of time.

A total inconvenience.

A kink in my plan.

A detour and distraction.

It's awful to accept and downright miserable to surrender to it.

And if you're a mom, it's almost impossible.

So there I was, thinking if I can only get this and that done, if I can make sure this was here and that was there, if I can manage a survival plan for my kids...

Then I would allow myself to rest.

Ugh.

So I plopped on my bed in such pain I couldn't find comfort in my soft pillow and supple sheets. I tossed and turned in a fatigue-induced fury. I agonized over what I could and should be doing with this restless time...

And then it hit me.

(God has a way of pouring a good dose of conviction right into my pity parties.)

I heard Him whisper…

> "This is temporary. Pray for those who endure
> longsuffering."

Gasp.

I lay still in silent surrender. My frenzied mind stopped, and my thoughts turned to each person I know who suffers agonizing days without end. My angst immediately transformed into a passionate prayer, as I named each precious soul I know who is held captive by some medical ailment or another. I pleaded for God to provide strength for them and their families. I begged for His healing. I lifted up every name I could think of and added those I don't know personally to the list. My heart was heavy and my eyes wet from weeping.

I used my pain for a purpose.

From now on, when I am ill or injured and need to rest… I will realize that the time I offer up in prayer for people in pain is truly time well spent.

Prayer is very productive. I can always show up for that.

6
HONOR YOUR HEALING

THERE WILL COME a time in your recovery when you will become impatient. *Why is it taking so long to heal?* Perhaps you didn't expect this to be so painful, or you surely didn't anticipate how long it would take to feel better. Maybe you were given a timeline and you aren't reaching those goals as easily as you thought you would. Worse yet, maybe you have been told that your recovery would be longer than the doctor originally anticipated. This is the hardest part of healing. I, for one, never experienced a nice, neat healing process. Not once. I've learned you really need to expect the unexpected.

Whether you are bedridden with illness or recovering from surgery or injury, healing takes more time than you ever think it will. This is the truth and one you must embrace. You may be so frustrated at this point that you force the recovery and push yourself more and more, only to find this doesn't work as you had hoped and now you are sore, weak, and exhausted. You might end up delaying your healing process even longer. I remember having my foot in a boot and wobbling down the stairs of a church to go teach my classes. I ended up falling, and I knew I damaged any healing that had already occurred as I hit my foot hard on the concrete step. And the **pain**. *Oh, the pain!* I pushed too hard too quickly and ended up falling back into the early stages of healing all over again. It was a disaster.

> *Please don't push it. This is the time in your life when you must surrender to the process and honor your healing. You must.*

You wake up each day with the hope you will be better than the day before, and sometimes you might be! On other days, you may feel the same or even worse.

Please be good to yourself. Your body needs your tender love and care to heal, and your mind is a powerful tool you can use either to promote healing or to sabotage it. When your thoughts turn critical, anxious, angry, or discouraged, it translates into your physical presence as well. What always helped me was to think of someone I love being in the same position. Would I speak to that person in the same way I talk to myself? Would I be impatient, uncaring, and critical of that beloved friend or family member? Be careful how you treat yourself these days, my friend. Pour grace onto every single struggle and tiny step forward. Train yourself in patience and acceptance. Respect your body and all it must do to completely recover. You cannot compare your pain and healing journey with that of anyone else. Even people with the same injury, surgery, or illness will recover differently. Just as you are made unique in your own extraordinary gifts and appearance, your body will heal in its own individualized way.

> *There is no right way to heal.*

This honoring process is extremely challenging. I know. For days, sometimes weeks—even months!—I would lament all the things I should have been doing. It's hard when you repeatedly fall short of your own expectations. You are so good at functioning nonstop every day that when you are forced to **stop** productivity, you can struggle with your sense of self-worth. You want to get things **done**, don't you? Yeah. I know. And there is so much **to do**, isn't there? Yeah. I get it. And you can't do **any** of those things that are swirling through your mind, driving you to the brink of insanity, depression, and escalating anxiety. Yep. Been there.

Here's the thing:

You need to love yourself **right** where you're at.

Being stripped of purpose, activity, and life as you once knew it to be can surely break open the ground you've built your identity upon and swallow you up. Perhaps you feel *"less than," "broken,"* or *"worthless"* while you wait to gain your ground once again. **This is not okay.** You cannot treat yourself like a failure or give up on who you are, simply because you aren't celebrating success or accomplishing all the things you once did. You must love yourself unconditionally, and if this is the lesson you learn through it all—

Then you have learned one of the greatest lessons in life.

I can testify to this very truth.

You will be forced either to love and accept yourself, or to hate and condemn yourself.

Please don't choose the latter. You deserve love, patience, compassion, and grace—now more than ever.

> *You have a choice every single day to honor who you are and how you are healing.*

The following exercise will help you find your worth in what may feel like wreckage. Instead of wallowing in all the things you cannot do and the ways you feel you are failing, how about you focus on those things you *can* do and celebrate that? You are not without purpose in who you are and what you can do. We've established many ways for you to discover that truth, and I want you to find more!

Don't forget who you are and how you are still being used for good. Let's explore your gifts, shall we?

What Are Your Gifts?

List all the gifts you have that you love.

Example

1. I love that I have a mind for statistics and numbers.
2. I love that I am a good mother.
3. I love the compassion I have for others.

1. _____

2. _____

3. _____

4. _____

5. _____

6. _____

7. _____

8. _____

9. _____

10. _____

How Can You Use These Gifts?

Connect a purpose to each gift.

Example

1. I can help my husband out with the bills.
2. I can snuggle with my kids and read to them.
3. I can be a prayer warrior for my church.

1. _____

2. _____

3. _____

4. _____

5. _____

6. _____

7. _____

8. _____

9. _____

10. _____

You Are Beautiful

Do you know that you are beautiful?
You are.
You were knitted together with His Divine Power.
Each thread is woven perfectly together to create
You.

Every fiber of your being
Is wonderfully and fearfully made.
Every piece and part of who you are
Is beautiful.

Your smile is like no other.
Your laughter. Your eyes. Your presence.
Your thoughts. Your dreams. Your fears.
All uniquely yours.

Your pain. Your story. Your battle. Your strength.
All beautiful.

Your passion. Your purpose.
Written before your days.
Your tears. Your dreams. Your soul.
Beautiful.

In the quiet moments when you weep,
God sees you.

In the silent night when you are alone,
Wondering, wishing, wavering,
Your thoughts are always precious to Him.
Your ways. Your secrets. Your soul.

He knows you.

He made you.

Beautiful you.

Every day has been ordained by Him.
He knows your path.
He knows your plan.
You're beautiful to Him.

So beautiful.

You have power.
You hold light.
You are the only you.
Beautiful.

Reach in deep.
Embrace your beauty.
The God of creation
Loves you.

Every piece of you.

Every detail and every deed.

Even the weakest part of you
Is beautiful.

You are beautiful.

Beautiful.

Beautiful.

Beautiful.

Honor Your Healing

His Workmanship is wonderful

In you.

Psalm 139:14

I praise you, for I am fearfully and wonderfully made. Wonderful are your works; my soul knows it very well.

7
ADJUST YOUR LENS

WHEN WE ARE suffering and stuck in stillness, our perspective shifts and shrinks to tunnel vision. We tighten our focus on the pain in the moment, and our mindset is limited to that small and narrow picture before us. We must be intentional with our thoughts and expand our vision to include the full scenery we are leaving out. It's so easy to lose sight of the big picture during these days full of tending to our wounds and our day-to-day tasks, simply surviving in the minutiae of it all.

It's time to adjust your lens. Open up your perspective, and break out of the barriers in which you feel bound. This period of your life can be used for reflection on your past tests and triumphs as you remember trials you overcame. You can stroll down memory lane, remembering when you celebrated success or took on specific challenges; you can relive moments when you felt empowered and strong. You can identify all the areas of your life that are fulfilling and feel gratitude despite your situation. You can embrace that which is significant and worthy of your acknowledgement and praise.

Widen your lens, expanding your thoughts to include the big picture. Your life is not defined by this season, nor will it ever be. The terrain is full of past and future hopes, dreams, and opportunities you continue to possess even while you are stuck waiting to live more completely again.

> *I finally discovered that if you can broaden your view—*
> *expanding the moments when your vision seems stuck—*
> *a massive shift in perspective happens.*

Are you bedridden? Take the focus off your aching body, wounds, or illness, and start turning that lens.

What is significant about your bedroom? What about any other rooms in your home?

When did you buy or rent the home you live in now? What's the story behind that?

Where do you plan to live many years from now? Where did you live before you moved into this home?

Who lives in your home with you? Are there memories in any of those rooms? Reflect on each room and the memories that bring you joy.

What about your family? What do they mean to you? Maybe each member of your family can bring you new snapshots and a collage of lovely views to take in.

Are there moments you want to treasure forever? Triumphs you have witnessed with your loved ones, or trials you have seen them through?

Are you looking forward to future events, trips, or celebrations?

The lens can be widened multiple times into rich, elaborate screenshots showcasing the magnificent scenery of your life.

Go there. Stick around and wander through past memories and future dreams. Rise high to take in the entire scope of the remarkable life you live. Tour your past accomplishments, visiting those stops along the way, reveling in this large map you own, full of so many lines, dots, and symbols reflecting the magnitude of the landscape before you.

Take it all in, friends. You can still enjoy your trip even while you're at this rest stop.

> *When we are healthier, in our fast-paced lifestyles, we often forget to embrace and reflect on the whole story. We may have missed some great views in our hurried pace. This can be our best opportunity to really take it all in.*

I'm betting you have quite a roadmap to open and trace in your mind. Enjoy the journey away from the place you are in now—

There are extraordinary stops along the way!

Shift Your Lens to a Wider Perspective

Perspective saves me.

I have written a lot about gratitude and the shift in how we look at things in our lives to find deeper meaning and purpose.

Something happens in your life, and you respond. You can either glance at it and carry on, or take the lens and twist it into focus. You can look deeper into the circumstance and discover many revelations as you grow in wisdom from such introspection. Embrace the moment, I say. Dwell in the depths of it.

I do that a lot.

I'm a thinker. And a feeler. And I respond.

But the perspective I'm working on is very different—and yet the same. Instead of focusing the lens closer, like a microscope studying the very specific situation and all the parts and pieces that belong to it...

I twist that lens wider to cover the landscape that carries the picture I am in. When I do that, I see more. I take in more. My focus expands to a much more significant scene that lifts me out of the magnified situation, pulling me farther away from it and shooting the larger picture.

Perspective.

*Often when I find myself in a crisis, or some difficult experience, I lunge hard and fast right into it without pulling back first. It takes intention to stop the lens from tightening into that initial image of what transpired and what could possibly come from it. We can lose ourselves right there in the thick of the frame. But if we can brace ourselves, and turn that lens back further to reveal the entire landscape surrounding that moment, we just might view it differently. We might **respond** differently, too.*

I have been in pain for about a month since the surgery on my foot and ankle. My life came to a jolted halt without the use of my leg. It's quite difficult getting around on one leg, ya know? I managed to fall pretty hard, spilling over myself and onto a bench in the hallway just this morning. Ouch. It's also difficult to run a household and care for children and surely impossible to drive school routes and run errands. I have dropped the ball on writing deadlines and book reviews. I also have taken the absentee role in various events and gatherings. "Rest and elevate" is the treatment while in my cast. I don't do either well. I've had to give up pretty much everything—at least it feels that way.

It's been a bit torturous.

I've had my meltdowns. I've sworn like a sailor and cried like a baby. I've pulled my big girl pants up and composed myself enough to "mother" from the couch and engage whenever I can with others. I've prayed for many people and challenged myself to think deeper to find significance and meaning behind—and beyond—this situation.

That's all fine and good, my usual way to cope with an unfortunate circumstance, but I realize there is something even more powerful to help change my perspective. I practice it quite often. I don't think I have described it before,

> *this expansion of my lens…*

Let me explain.

I feel the pain.

My lens was magnified intensely on that focal point when I swore and whined.

*But if I stretch the lens a bit further out, you would find my family surrounding me with helping hands and serving hearts when I am in need. You'd see the mess of a home without the "homemaker," but you would see the dishes done and the laundry folded and the **most important** things completed by my husband and friends who come by with meals and a helping hand. Stretch that lens further out…*

*You would watch me playing a game of ball in the summer sun, laughing and embracing time with family as I so carefully placed cones on the divots in the yard, promising to **not** twist my ankle. Running to first base, I went down. But stretch further, and you will see a weekend of love and laughter and the beautiful new land my sister lives on, where our children played half-naked with their cousins in the flowing creek and the acres of woods. You would be warmed by the campfire and wooed by the s'mores. Ah, the memories...*

Twist again to widen the scope...

You would discover 30 years of walking in pain—and the revelation that finally something has been done about it! You would realize this is the beginning of a new way to walk and a path to freedom, thanks to some incredible doctors and their expertise. I am blessed to have the option of being "fixed."

Wind that lens still more...

You would see a beautiful home, loving "get well" cards, and people calling, sending texts, or stopping by to check on me. You would find a community full of organizations, resources, and people—one in which we are blessed to belong. Stretch that lens further and you will span the country and beyond to beloved friends and writers I adore connecting with through the web. You would discover family members who send special gifts, cards, and loving prayers for my healing. Twist the lens forward, and you will go beyond January and into February, where I will be without a cast and in a new boot going to physical therapy to learn how to walk again. Tweak the lens one more time to span May and June, which are full of new life, warmer days, and me taking long walks reflecting on a winter of stillness and pain but feeling so grateful for my recovery.

When the lens gets bigger, the dire situation gets smaller.

Expand your lens. Open your borders. Stretch your frame. The surrounding scenery may enhance the picture, and the landscape may add an entirely new dimension to your focal point. When difficulties happen, we naturally zoom in on the circumstances. Sometimes we allow them to take over the bigger picture.

Don't zoom in too long, or you may lose the power of the big-picture perspective.

Stretch it out.

Pull further away to survey the scope of it all.

Change the frame.

Enlarge the landscape.

Wider.

Wider.

Even wider—

Until you reach your best shot.

The new scenery will surely change the view.

8

Own It, Laugh a Little, and Get Out!

HERE'S THE THING: You are physically broken right now.

You might not have showered for days, and the stench you exude proves it. Perhaps you can't make yourself "look well" even if you try. You may be in a cast or using a walker or motorized scooter. You may be in a sling or neck brace, possibly even a wheelchair. Have you crawled on the floor to get to the bathroom or worn clothes that barely cover parts you'd rather have hidden? Do you have sores in places that don't see the light of day? Maybe there are newly formed scars appearing that look horrific, or you are trying to accept new renovations to your body that don't compare to the body you had before. You might look like a mangled mess. You've gone from a functioning, put-together class act to feeling like a greasy, no-make-up, stinky, unkempt misfit. I'm betting you are feeling vulnerable and insecure about this body of yours and how it looks and functions. Being broken can be humiliating, am I right? Being exposed, dependent, and weak can add layers of shame and embarrassment. I know. This broken business is brutal and often humiliating.

This is where you must simply *own it*. You are human, and every single human being on this earth has been, or will be, broken at some point in his or her life. Your body is a miraculous blend of precious parts and pieces that deserve honor and respect from you.

Remember always: Not one person has it all together. *Not one.*

You need to be okay with where you're at right now. You should embrace your body and lift your head with confidence.

The greatest challenge is when you are out in public. People stare. With each set of eyes watching you, your self-worth can crumble, and you may want to escape the scene as quickly as your broken body will allow. Maybe your pride is battered, knowing that others look on you with compassion. For me, the worst part of any recovery was noticing people getting frustrated with my inability to rush or move at their pace. The pressure can be unbearable, and you may be tempted to give up on getting out of the house.

> *It's easier to stay put in the comfort of your own home.*
> *Don't.*

You **need** to get out. If this means having a friend assist you, ask them. If this means you can drive to the nearest store to simply pick up some milk, do it. If it means people will stare, sigh, or make statements that aren't kind—so be it. Think of places where you feel the most comfortable. Maybe it's the library or even simply having a friend take you for a drive.

After my friend had surgery, she was laid up for weeks. I invited her along on my carpool rides, picking up several kids at three different schools and taking them all home. Every day, I picked her up first and she rode along in the front of the car as we laughed and talked. This was her way of engaging and connecting with the world from her own comfort zone—my car. What was most important was that she was able to leave her home and take in new scenery, enjoying face-to-face interactions while coming along for the ride. She got *out*.

Do it. I promise you, it will be worth the effort preparing and planning for an outing. It may take an hour to dress and another hour to get in the car, but it will be worth every minute you are in a fresh, new environment. Your senses and spirit will thank you.

I learned to take the outings on with confidence because when you exude that, something shifts in the atmosphere around you. Acknowledge your limitations with lighthearted comments or funny jokes! Tell people to go around you when there is impatience. Start conversations with others without feeling uncomfortable in your own skin. Smile. Yes, *smile*. Look people in the eyes and smile, even when you look and feel like a hot mess.

> *It's amazing what a smile can do for you and the recipient.*

I hated being handicapped—every single time I had surgery. I hated not being able to get around like I used to with ease and speed, so I often made it all a game. Whoever took me to the store witnessed the joy of having one crazy friend run the mobilized cart into displays, yell, "Look out!" at complete strangers, and back up with that annoying *beep, beep, beep* just to make that sound over and over again. People stared. They sighed. But I laughed. I laughed at myself and hammed it up every time.

My situation felt ridiculous, pathetic, and downright embarrassing, so I ended up having a blast making fun of myself and embracing the awkward attention of onlookers. It helped to have a friend shaking her head and giggling while nervously trying to excuse my behavior. I would make jokes with strangers who looked at me with puzzling, uncertain gazes. I would let my kids ride along with me as they squealed, "Go *faster*, Mommy! *Faster*!"

My outings became fun despite the humiliation because I proactively decided I was going to *own it* and laugh a little along the way.

What have you got to lose?

> *I think we all can pull off a bit of comic relief—no matter what we're going through.*

My friend, I know that what you are experiencing is difficult, painful, and incredibly frustrating. I promise a little laughter will lift you, and we all could use a lift during our recovery.

If you have been stuck in one spot, take courage and step out into a new scene. Accept that you may get looks, groans, complaints, or even questions. Take on the challenge with a new sense of pride, and always remember that every single person out there will, at some point in his or her life, be broken. So *have no shame*. If you are unable to get out by yourself, call a helper from your contact list and ask if someone can escort you on an outing: a drive, a visit to someone's house, a movie, or even simply going through a drive-through for some greasy fries and a shake.

It will be worth the work and will make a huge difference in your well-being.

Do it, okay?

Find the *fun*.

It's there—in you.

Funny Can Be Found Anywhere

I suppose people would call me an "inspirational writer," but little do they know, in real life, I am a hilarious fool. I am! I love making people laugh with my crazy, incessant ways. Ask anyone I know, and she will surely have a few stories about me cracking the boundaries of appropriateness somewhere. It's who I am. I wish sometimes I could push through the screen of my laptop and show the world that side of me—but I will share my twisted humor here instead.

After finding out my sister had Stage III breast cancer, I succumbed to her desperate wishes for me to be tested for the genetic mutation. After she was found to be BRCA1 positive, she worried about her sisters having the same mutation, which would result in an almost 90 percent risk of following in her footsteps. Other factors in our history pointed to the inevitable: Our mother's mother died at an early age of breast cancer, and I already had abnormal growths watched closely through quarterly ultrasounds as a result of two biopsies. It was time I respected my sister's wishes and got tested.

I had the BRCA1 mutation.

After months of multiple doctor visits, tests, and pre-op assessments, I made some life-changing decisions. I ended up at the hospital one cold December morning being prepped for the excavation of all my woman parts. Yes. I was facing three surgeons with three surgeries all in one:

>*a double mastectomy, breast reconstruction, and a full hysterectomy...*

>*at the tender age of 43 years old.*

It was a brutal season. My precious daughter was struggling with ongoing debilitating medical issues, which left me suffocating with despair and living with little sleep, all the while enduring pre-op appointments with both my three- and six-year-old kids strapped to my side. During this time, my husband traveled for business, so I spent two months navigating this path by myself.

It's amazing how strength finds its way to you when you least expect it.

One thing I know for sure is that there is always light in laughter, and we must uncover it even in the darkest moments of our lives. There are highlights threaded throughout this story that reveal just that—a bit of shining laughter where you would, once again, least expect it.

My very first appointment to find out what on earth I should do with this BRCA1 mutation was with a breast surgeon who would later remove my breasts. I was terrified. My dear friend came with me to take notes. I sat there topless with the paper gown wrapped tightly around me, anxiously waiting for what seemed like hours. When she entered the room, she seemed detached and stoic, which made me even more nervous. As she looked at her clipboard and went through the typical introductions, she motioned for me to place "them" on the tray. Little did I know she meant the papers I had in my hands! I went over and began to open my wrap and awkwardly place my breasts on the tray! She immediately corrected me, and from that moment on, I realized this was going to be one heck of a ride!

(You can laugh now. It's freaking funny!)

*Fast-forward through the medical twists and turns of this story to the pre-op room at dawn that dreaded morning. As the surgeons and nurses roamed the area preparing for the surgery, I sat there shivering naked under the hospital gown—but with a huge hospital-sized pad on for my lovely period (the last one I would ever have—one silver lining **for sure***!). *The nurse finally found me, after what felt like forever, and fumbled around the tubes and tape to hook up my IV. She looked frazzled, and after reading the charts from all three surgeons, she seemed unable to manage it all. She nervously claimed I had too many surgeries for her to organize all the paperwork; apparently, her ankle was hurting since she woke up, and she couldn't even get around very well. I'm not sure if her incompetence was a gift or a curse, so I will let you decide.*

As she shared a tearful story of her son's untimely death, I entered "counselor mode" and talked her through some of her grief. I helped her sift through some of the layers of pain she had wrapped herself in, and

90

her demeanor began to lighten. After she expressed her gratitude to me for having helped her, I gently reminded her that there were still two more vials of blood to take lying empty on the tray next to me. Looking back, I am just glad she wasn't my surgeon! (Wow!)

*My breast surgeon came in to mark me where she would be cutting and carving around my chest, and I started to realize this was actually going to happen! After all the pre-op traffic died down, I sat there in silence, becoming more anxious while waiting for my husband to come in. When he was with me to say "goodbye," I asked him to grab some paper towels so I could wipe off the nervous sweat that had been dripping from my armpits down my sides. I stuffed them under my gown to dry my armpits and glanced at the towel to see **black ink**! I had smeared all the markings made by my surgeon!*

*I completely **lost it**!*

*Derek ran to get a nurse to find the surgeon before she disappeared into the operating room. I prayed she could fix this incomprehensible mess! I was humiliated and horrified, and yet, at the same time, I found this hilarious! I mean, are you **kidding me**? I seriously thought to myself: "Only **you**, Chrissy! Only **you**." The breast surgeon came in to take a close look at what I smeared and drew over the messy parts as I chuckled with a nervous gasp: "I can't believe I did that!"*

(I wonder if she ever sat around with other doctors sharing these ridiculous stories about me. I will never know.)

Surgery went well. There was high risk of infection with all three surgeries at the same time, but everything went as planned. (Thank You, God!)

The recovery was brutal. I can't lie. I couldn't move or even breathe without feeling great pain. My pectoral muscles were so tight that I couldn't pull my shoulders back to get air into my lungs. I came out of this surgery bloated into a morbidly gruesome human being with bloody stitches and bruising like I had never seen before. It was awful! My sweet husband gave me a sponge bath every night while I whimpered in pain. I ended up having an infection in one breast, which left me with an additional dose of suffering.

One very important part of this story is that I was blessed with the most generous, amazing church family and incredible friends who were with me every step of the way. We had a cooler on our front porch for almost two months regularly filled with food, gifts, and encouraging notes every single day. **Every single day!** *I still look back and remember each beautiful person who stepped in. I will never forget them.*

The surgery was at the beginning of December 2009. Since I wouldn't be sending Christmas cards out that year, and I hardly saw a soul all season, I wanted to write a heartfelt letter of thanks to all the people who loved and cared for our family during that time. I figured that while I was at it, I would send the same letter to everyone on our Christmas card list as well. Why not?

At the end of my message, I decided it was time to own it and laugh a little. I wrote that I was betting they were curious what my new breasts looked like. With that last line, I shared a photo of a woman in a seductive top barely covering her voluptuous breasts! I sent the same letter to friends and family thanking them for their support—with the added note and picture at the end.

Let me tell you, I still laugh until I cry with that zinger! My best friend from high school mentioned it years later and said, "Only **you** *could pull that off, Chrissy!"*

[In its original form, this article was originally published at Menopausal Mother (www.menopausalmom.com) on Tuesday, January 28, 2014.]

9
PRAYER AND SPIRITUALITY

WHILE YOU WAIT for your life to carry on, this time you are on *"hold"* can be an important period of reflection, awareness, and discovery. You may even learn a few things about yourself you never knew! I know I did.

Religion/spirituality is a significant part of many people's lives. This is one area that should not be neglected, especially now. Whatever you believe, however and whomever you worship, I encourage you to dive deeply into this place of faith. For me, Christ is the only answer and true source of peace.

I cannot speak to the many various religions out there, so if you practice a faith other than Christianity, I want to support you in your healing, no matter what your spiritual direction is.

If you are not affiliated with any religion, but you have always wondered about a particular area of faith—this is the time to investigate and explore! Ask God to reveal Himself to you.

If you don't care to seek God, I urge you to find comfort in other practices I haven't mentioned in this book. Whatever brings you peace in your life, I hope you are able to dig deeper into ***that***.

If you are a woman of the Christian faith, prayer and the power of God's Word (the Bible) can surely offer you comfort, nourishment, and hope. During all my recovery times, I was in constant prayer asking God to grow me and open up new parts of me He wanted to tend to, edify, and sanctify. If you read the Bible, there is plenty of food for your soul as well as practical wisdom. It truly is a timeless manual for every part of life. In living through what might seem like an empty desert, this is the perfect time to dive into the Word of God to find comfort and strength in scripture.

Perhaps God wants to reveal something new to you about yourself and your relationship with Him. If you listen carefully, He may show Himself to you in an entirely new way.

> *This may be the first time God has had you all to Himself, and if you allow the stillness to be a place of sacred solace, there may be great fruit to come from it!*

There are endless books you can read that can guide you through biblical wisdom and the power of God's Word in your life. There are devotionals that can help you focus on your prayer life while discovering God's presence in your quiet moments. I believe God's plan for you is full of ***hope*** and ***purpose***. This season is in His hands—if you let Him take it. There are no moments wasted in His plan. You can offer your time and your heart to Him, and He will gladly take them and bless you with something miraculous.

You may not know how to pray. That's okay! If my words spark an interest for you, then let me share the most useful prayer equation I've come to know.

94

Philippians 4:6-8 helps me walk through a simple prayer I often use with God.

Philippians 4:6-8

Do not be anxious about anything, but in everything by prayer and supplication with thanksgiving let your requests be made known to God.

And the peace of God, which surpasses all understanding, will guard your hearts and your minds in Christ Jesus.

Finally, brothers, whatever is true, whatever is honorable, whatever is just, whatever is pure, whatever is lovely, whatever is commendable, if there is any excellence, if there is anything worthy of praise, think about these things.

Four-Step Prayer

1. Tell God what you are feeling and what you need.

2. Thank God for all you have.

3. Trust that God will bring you peace in all those areas you offered to Him.

4. Keep your thoughts on all good things.

My friends, please understand this: *Prayer is simply talking to God.*

There is **no** right way to approach Him. He created you; therefore, He already knows your heart and your thoughts. You can be exactly **you** when you pray. You don't need a biblical degree. You don't have to go to a church to pray. You don't have to say specific things or feel certain feelings. You don't even have to have more than a morsel of faith.

> *One thing is for sure: God deeply loves you and wants so desperately to hear from you.*

Go to Him.

He will offer you grace, comfort, peace, wisdom, assurance, confidence, forgiveness, purpose, counsel, and hope. You simply have to ask Him for it.

Step 1: Tell God what you are feeling and what you need.

What is on your heart? What troubles, challenges, or upsets you? Lay it all out there, girls. Let it *go*...

God, my heart hurts. I'm scared. I don't feel loved by my mom, or the rest of the family. I'm scared about the state of my health. I feel a lot of regret for all of my mistakes. I'm hurt that I don't feel seen or accepted for who I am by my family. I want to be vibrantly healthy and happy.

Step 2: Thank God for all you have.

What are you able to thank God for in your life? Let your mind scan all the areas you have spent time writing down in previous chapters. Reflect on it all, and thank God for each and every one of those areas you enjoy. Perhaps you can identify previously answered prayers and thank God for those as well.

Thank you God for giving me a second chance at life. Thank you God for Anastasia, Lyzzi, and Morgan. Thank you God for providing me with shelter and food to eat. Thank you God for healing my injuries in the best ways possible and for my bone graft being successful.

Step 3: Trust that God will bring you peace in all the areas you offered to Him.

Find peace in knowing God now has it all in His hands and He will work all things to the good of those who love Him (Romans 8:28). Take this quiet prayer time to allow God to minister to your heart. Trust that He will bring you peace. It's okay if you don't *feel* that peace right away. Everyone experiences peace differently and in a different time frame. At times, I have waited months before peace fully took hold of my heart, so don't be discouraged if you still feel anguish even after your prayer. Trust that peace will come.

Step 4: Keep your thoughts on all good things.

Continue to focus on what is worthy of praise! Remind yourself of all those blessings in your life that still continue to give you joy, laughter, peace, and love. **Look at your gratitude list!** You can scribble your thoughts here to keep them fresh in your mind.

I am so looking forward to having my own place (with a trustworthy roommate) and with Oscar, more kitties and doggies—I can't wait to have a dog! I just want a home full of love and animals, somewhere warm and close to the beach. A life filled with beaching, yoga, smoothies, green juice, friends, pets, and finally love.

*If you are interested in learning more about Christianity, in addition to the Bible, I encourage you to read any of these books:

- *The Case for Christ* by Lee Strobel
- *The Case for a Creator* by Lee Strobel
- *Mere Christianity* by C.S. Lewis
- *Jesus the One and Only* by Beth Moore
- *No Wonder They Call Him the Savior* by Max Lucado (or **anything** by him)
- *The Purpose Driven Life: What on Earth Am I Here For?* by Rick Warren

To Walk in Faith...

One foot trembles, as it taps on the water.
The drops wet my skin, and I'm scared I will falter.
I stand on the boat, as it sways back and forth...
To the rhythm of the waves...
In the sun-drenched haze.

"Come," You say.
"Lord, how?" I pray.
"Believe!" You cry.
"I'm trying!" I lie.

I stare out at the others
Splashing in the sea,
Desperately doubting—
I see parts of me.

"What if I fall?"
I question again.
"Trust in My power."
He reached out His hand.

"I'd much rather trust You
On shore where it's safe."

"But My way is best
For your own sake."

"I know, I know...
But it's easier here.
Could You just come closer?
I must feel You near."

"Oh, child, dear child,
Such faith you lack!"

"I'm sorry, so sorry.
I'll turn the boat back."

"Please don't do that.
This way is My plan.
Just take those first steps;
You'll see who I Am."

I shake and I shiver.
I know what to do.
"But I fear that the wind
Might blind me from You."

"Your eyes stay on Me.
That is the key.
Stop frantically fretting
So anxiously.

"Stop waiting and wondering
And worrying how.
Your battle is over.
I've got you now.

"Take that first step and
Reach out to Me.
Stop trying so hard.
Don't look at the sea!"

"Come," You say.
"Come walk to Me."

I splatter and crash
Into waves that I pass.
The wind blinds my eyes,
But I know they are lies.

One step at a time,
I don't lose His gaze,
My eyes fixed on Him
In the sun-drenched haze.

Matthew 14:28-31

And Peter answered him,
"Lord, if it is you, command me to come to you on the water."
He said, "Come."
So Peter got out of the boat and walked on the water and came to
Jesus.
But when he saw the wind, he was afraid, and beginning to sink
he cried out, "Lord, save me."
Jesus immediately reached out his hand and took hold of him,
saying to him,
"O you of little faith, why did you doubt?"

One step at a time,
I walk in faith.

10
A NEW DAY

WHEREVER YOU ARE on this healing journey, I want to promise you something:

There will be a day when you are done healing.

There **will** be a day when you are back into life full swing, your body will be working again, and you will be recovered! It may look different from what you planned. A limp here, a limitation there, perhaps some changes have been made to your lifestyle in some way, due to injury, surgery, or illness. Perhaps you won't have any remaining hints of this season and your life will carry on with this tiny blip on your timeline already fading fast.

Let me give you hope!

One day you will be doing chores or hosting a dinner party, and you will realize you couldn't do that last year because you were so sick. Maybe you will be at the gym when it hits you just how far you have come since that injury. Perhaps you'll find yourself gazing at your scars while in the shower and nodding to yourself with wonder at all you've been through and how hard it was. You may even tear up thinking about how hopeless or grueling your recovery seemed.

Maybe you'll giggle at all the crawling you had to do on the floor or how you always ran your motorized scooter into displays at the grocery store.

Perhaps you will find this book with your scribbles on it and reflect on the growth you gained from the experience. Each day further out from this difficult season, you will discover more to celebrate, appreciate, and commemorate. There will be **great joy** in your new awareness and appreciation of being healthy and whole. There will be immeasurable gratitude for regaining your strength and vitality.

And most of all?

> *You will have a new segment on your timeline that has been filled with fresh inspiration, new wisdom, and perhaps deeper faith.*

You will treasure what you discovered during the long, quiet moments of reflection, dreaming, and digging deep to find passion, purpose, and new ideas for the road ahead. You will be able to give back and enjoy the blessing of serving others, knowing how it feels to be cared for and loved.

You might even shift your agenda and focus after realizing there are some things you can eliminate from your life. There may be things you want to add. You may even take some significant turns in your career or make much-needed changes with your free time after learning additional hobbies, realizing new interests, or discovering fresh priorities that could have only come from that time "*off.*" Maybe you grew deeper in your faith, sparking a desire to seek out a place of worship. Perhaps you have created goals for a newly inspired passion because you were able to identify something worth pursuing.

> *Your life will be changed. Your life will be richer—for having survived being broken.*

Some things need to be broken, opened, and taken apart to let light in.

Look for the light, my friend. It is shining somewhere in you.

I promise.

Beauty Blooms in Hard Places

Hard places,
Life's messes

Can suffocate the hope
Right out of us—

If we let them.

Stuck
Under the heavy weight

Of barriers and barricades,
Hurling bombs and blown grenades.

We squirm, we sweat,
We reach, we stretch,
We grab, we groan,
We claw at stone.

And we are forced to do hard things
In hard places.

Hard places,
Life's messes:
They hurt.

A New Day

But beauty blooms
In hard places.

Beauty blooms
In life's messes.

Behold!
Do you see?
It's glorious.

Unearthed strength from where you lie,
Rising vibrant colors fly
From broken, buried, battered, bruised

Comes
Healing, wholeness, hope
In you.

11
AND ANOTHER THING...

AFTER YOU ARE all healed and life has returned to its rapid pace, you may still have those lovely little reminders of this difficult season: that twinge of pain comes along now and again, or maybe your arm doesn't quite boast the strength it once did. Perhaps you are on new medication that has recurring side effects you have to manage, or you have limitations on your body that you didn't have before. I continue to feel reminders all the time.

And you know what? I'm glad I do. And you should be glad too.

> *Those reminders of healing may always linger, and I'd like to think of them as gracious blessings.*

They are, in fact, part of who you are, who I am. And if you can look back and realize the strength you found while bearing through the healing process, despite all the time and effort it took to get you to this place—it's **worth it**! It's all worth it because, if you are like me, you learned so much along the way. You discovered things about yourself that you didn't know, or you possibly learned how to let go and receive help from others. I bet you figured out that the world doesn't stop spinning once you do, but that people show up to keep it moving along after all. Your children may have proven to be amazingly patient and helpful, or you came to the conclusion that you needed to adjust your priorities to fit your interests and activities. Whatever gifts you opened through this experience are invaluable, and you can pass them on to a loved one when they find themselves stuck in the season of stillness, too. Maybe you have unearthed a grand garden of gratitude that you have learned to cultivate regularly, finding more meaning in your day-to-day life.

If anything, you are surely glad to be healed—however that may look.

May I remind you of the greatest lesson you learned during this time?

> *You've proved to yourself that you can overcome obstacles.*

You've come through it. You've survived. You've managed to make it.

So when those reminders linger on in your day, your *life*—

Think of them as reminders that you are *here.*

You are *alive*, and you are something special.

I hope they never let you forget it.

Your Pain Is a Beautiful Reminder

I was lying in bed in pain the other night. Everything that was ever broken in me was wide awake and swarming my body with reminders. I was still nauseous and aching from another accidental gluten ingestion. My ear was burning and twitching, my breasts burst with that familiar sharp surge, and my foot was flooded with a stinging current ripping through my joint. I felt the various pains rise and fall over and over again while my mind followed them and tightly wound around each one. Here I was again, receiving the echoes of past surgeries, injuries, and an illness that still lingered without my control. My sleep was delayed by the hurting hints of recovery.

As I retraced the pain, I found myself wandering through the memories of each circumstance, unwinding those tight grips of thought and slowly threading a new resolve within.

"These are my reminders," I said to myself.

And with that thought poured forth the realization of the deep gratitude I hold for each and every one of them.

Although my nerve is affected by taking out a tumor, how blessed I am that it was benign!

Although new breasts still refuse to accept their place, I thank God I do not have breast cancer!

Although my feet will never be without pain, I am still able to use them efficiently and remarkably so!

Although I still battle chronic illness at the time of this writing, I am grateful for newfound solutions to help me heal and am hopeful more answers will come.

These are my reminders. And each time I experience a familiar pain, I offer up praise and celebration instead of discouragement and disdain. Am I not blessed with new insights, answers, interventions, and outcomes, all of which keep graciously growing me into who I am today?

Am I not grateful to be alive and well enough to live a life of great fulfillment and abundant joy, all unique to my journey?

How on earth do I begrudge that?

Never again.

I don't want these reminders to ever fade away…I want to embrace the sorely significant truth that I, in fact, am still here remembering.

I never want to forget.

If I forgot, I wouldn't be reminded over and over again to take a closer look at those memories and settle the pain in purpose. To live with each sting, jab, and ache reminds me that I am alive and there is a reason for it.

Yes. I thank God for reminding me always how blessed I truly am.

Are there places of pain that linger in you? Oh, friends, if you are still here on this earth feeling them…

Then you need to celebrate your reminders, too.

ADDITIONAL NOTES

These pages are for you to fill with your thoughts, hopes, ideas, frustrations, or even drawings. I wanted to give you space to use in a way that is meaningful to you.

Christine would love to connect with you in the following ways:

The Mom Café Blog
www.themomcafe.com

Twitter
@themomcafe
twitter.com/themomcafe

Facebook
facebook.com/TheMomCafe

Pinterest
pinterest.com/themomcafe/

Email
Chris@TheMomCafe.com

Updates on future publications can be found at:

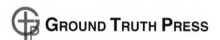 **GROUND TRUTH PRESS**

P.O. Box 7313
Nashua, NH 03060-7313

www.groundtruthpress.com

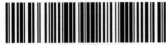

Made in the USA
Middletown, DE
12 November 2017